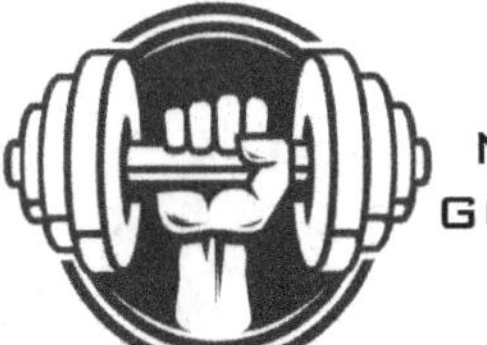

WORKOUT LOG

NAME: _______________
GOALS: _______________
DATE: _______________
STATS: _______________
WEIGHT: _______________

EXERCISE:	SETS	REPS	WEIGHT	REST	SETS	REPS	WEIGHT	REST	SETS	REPS	WEIGHT	REST	SETS	REPS	WEIGHT	REST

CARDIO:	TIME	DIST.	INT.	PACE	TIME	DIST.	INT.	PACE	TIME	DIST.	INT.	PACE	TIME	DIST.	INT.	PACE

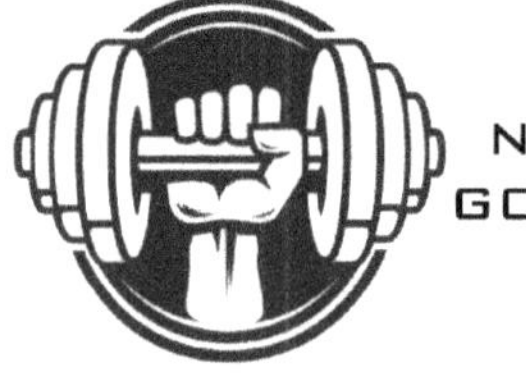

WORKOUT LOG

NAME: ______________________________________

GOALS: ______________________________________

DATE:

STATS:

WEIGHT:

EXERCISE:	SETS	REPS	WEIGHT	REST	SETS	REPS	WEIGHT	REST	SETS	REPS	WEIGHT	REST	SETS	REPS	WEIGHT	REST

CARDIO:	TIME	DIST.	INT.	PACE	TIME	DIST.	INT.	PACE	TIME	DIST.	INT.	PACE	TIME	DIST.	INT.	PACE

WORKOUT LOG

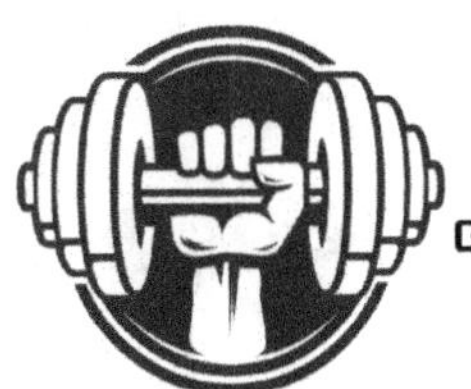

NAME: _______________________________

GOALS: _______________________________

DATE: ________ ________ ________ ________

STATS: ________ ________ ________ ________

WEIGHT: ________ ________ ________ ________

EXERCISE:	SETS	REPS	WEIGHT	REST	SETS	REPS	WEIGHT	REST	SETS	REPS	WEIGHT	REST	SETS	REPS	WEIGHT	REST

CARDIO:	TIME	DIST.	INT.	PACE	TIME	DIST.	INT.	PACE	TIME	DIST.	INT.	PACE	TIME	DIST.	INT.	PACE

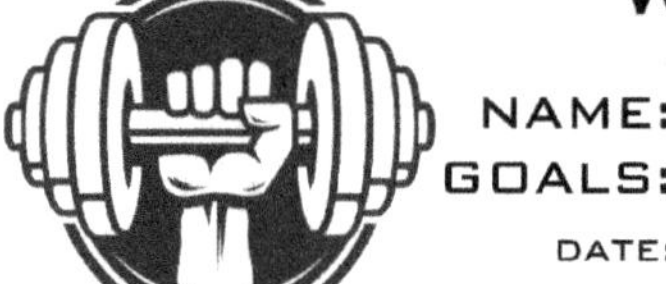

WORKOUT LOG

NAME:
GOALS:
DATE:
STATS:
WEIGHT:

EXERCISE:	SETS	REPS	WEIGHT	REST	SETS	REPS	WEIGHT	REST	SETS	REPS	WEIGHT	REST	SETS	REPS	WEIGHT	REST

CARDIO:	TIME	DIST.	INT.	PACE	TIME	DIST.	INT.	PACE	TIME	DIST.	INT.	PACE	TIME	DIST.	INT.	PACE

WORKOUT LOG

NAME:

GOALS:

DATE:

STATS:

WEIGHT:

EXERCISE:	SETS	REPS	WEIGHT	REST	SETS	REPS	WEIGHT	REST	SETS	REPS	WEIGHT	REST	SETS	REPS	WEIGHT	REST

CARDIO:	TIME	DIST.	INT.	PACE	TIME	DIST.	INT.	PACE	TIME	DIST.	INT.	PACE	TIME	DIST.	INT.	PACE

WORKOUT LOG

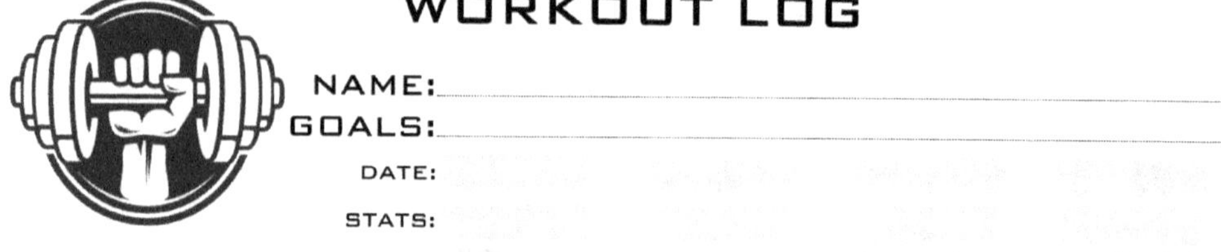

NAME:

GOALS:

DATE:

STATS:

WEIGHT:

EXERCISE:	SETS	REPS	WEIGHT	REST	SETS	REPS	WEIGHT	REST	SETS	REPS	WEIGHT	REST	SETS	REPS	WEIGHT	REST

CARDIO:	TIME	DIST.	INT.	PACE	TIME	DIST.	INT.	PACE	TIME	DIST.	INT.	PACE	TIME	DIST.	INT.	PACE

WORKOUT LOG

NAME:

GOALS:

DATE:

STATS:

WEIGHT:

EXERCISE:	SETS	REPS	WEIGHT	REST	SETS	REPS	WEIGHT	REST	SETS	REPS	WEIGHT	REST	SETS	REPS	WEIGHT	REST

CARDIO:	TIME	DIST.	INT.	PACE	TIME	DIST.	INT.	PACE	TIME	DIST.	INT.	PACE	TIME	DIST.	INT.	PACE

WORKOUT LOG

NAME:

GOALS:

DATE:

STATS:

WEIGHT:

EXERCISE:	SETS	REPS	WEIGHT	REST	SETS	REPS	WEIGHT	REST	SETS	REPS	WEIGHT	REST	SETS	REPS	WEIGHT	REST

CARDIO:	TIME	DIST.	INT.	PACE	TIME	DIST.	INT.	PACE	TIME	DIST.	INT.	PACE	TIME	DIST.	INT.	PACE

WORKOUT LOG

NAME:

GOALS:

DATE:

STATS:

WEIGHT:

EXERCISE:	SETS	REPS	WEIGHT	REST	SETS	REPS	WEIGHT	REST	SETS	REPS	WEIGHT	REST	SETS	REPS	WEIGHT	REST

CARDIO:	TIME	DIST.	INT.	PACE	TIME	DIST.	INT.	PACE	TIME	DIST.	INT.	PACE	TIME	DIST.	INT.	PACE

WORKOUT LOG

NAME:

GOALS:

DATE:

STATS:

WEIGHT:

EXERCISE:	SETS	REPS	WEIGHT	REST	SETS	REPS	WEIGHT	REST	SETS	REPS	WEIGHT	REST	SETS	REPS	WEIGHT	REST

CARDIO:	TIME	DIST.	INT.	PACE	TIME	DIST.	INT.	PACE	TIME	DIST.	INT.	PACE	TIME	DIST.	INT.	PACE

WORKOUT LOG

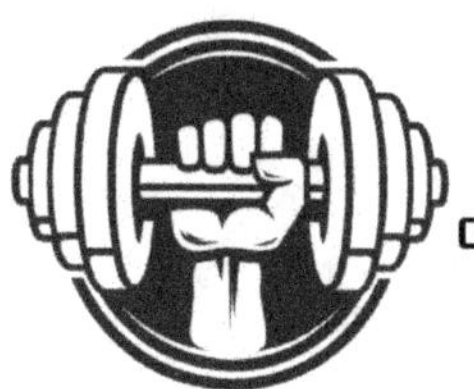

NAME:

GOALS:

DATE:

STATS:

WEIGHT:

EXERCISE:	SETS	REPS	WEIGHT	REST	SETS	REPS	WEIGHT	REST	SETS	REPS	WEIGHT	REST	SETS	REPS	WEIGHT	REST

CARDIO:	TIME	DIST.	INT.	PACE	TIME	DIST.	INT.	PACE	TIME	DIST.	INT.	PACE	TIME	DIST.	INT.	PACE

WORKOUT LOG

NAME:
GOALS:
DATE:
STATS:
WEIGHT:

EXERCISE:	SETS	REPS	WEIGHT	REST	SETS	REPS	WEIGHT	REST	SETS	REPS	WEIGHT	REST	SETS	REPS	WEIGHT	REST

CARDIO:	TIME	DIST.	INT.	PACE	TIME	DIST.	INT.	PACE	TIME	DIST.	INT.	PACE	TIME	DIST.	INT.	PACE

WORKOUT LOG

NAME:
GOALS:
DATE:
STATS:
WEIGHT:

EXERCISE:	SETS	REPS	WEIGHT	REST	SETS	REPS	WEIGHT	REST	SETS	REPS	WEIGHT	REST	SETS	REPS	WEIGHT	REST

CARDIO:	TIME	DIST.	INT.	PACE	TIME	DIST.	INT.	PACE	TIME	DIST.	INT.	PACE	TIME	DIST.	INT.	PACE

WORKOUT LOG

NAME:

GOALS:

DATE:

STATS:

WEIGHT:

EXERCISE:	SETS	REPS	WEIGHT	REST	SETS	REPS	WEIGHT	REST	SETS	REPS	WEIGHT	REST	SETS	REPS	WEIGHT	REST

CARDIO:	TIME	DIST.	INT.	PACE	TIME	DIST.	INT.	PACE	TIME	DIST.	INT.	PACE	TIME	DIST.	INT.	PACE

WORKOUT LOG

NAME:
GOALS:
DATE:
STATS:
WEIGHT:

EXERCISE:	SETS	REPS	WEIGHT	REST	SETS	REPS	WEIGHT	REST	SETS	REPS	WEIGHT	REST	SETS	REPS	WEIGHT	REST

CARDIO:	TIME	DIST.	INT.	PACE	TIME	DIST.	INT.	PACE	TIME	DIST.	INT.	PACE	TIME	DIST.	INT.	PACE

WORKOUT LOG

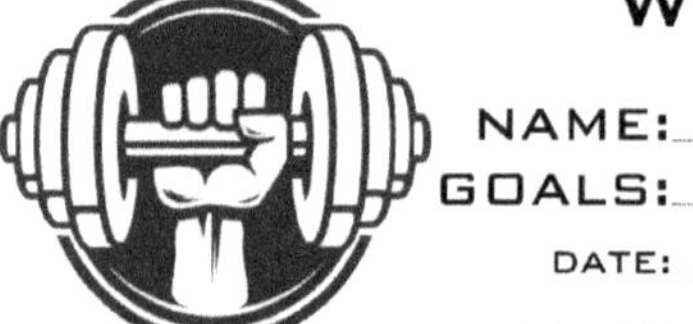

NAME:

GOALS:

DATE:

STATS:

WEIGHT:

EXERCISE:	SETS	REPS	WEIGHT	REST	SETS	REPS	WEIGHT	REST	SETS	REPS	WEIGHT	REST	SETS	REPS	WEIGHT	REST

CARDIO:	TIME	DIST.	INT.	PACE	TIME	DIST.	INT.	PACE	TIME	DIST.	INT.	PACE	TIME	DIST.	INT.	PACE

WORKOUT LOG

NAME:

GOALS:

DATE:

STATS:

WEIGHT:

EXERCISE:	SETS	REPS	WEIGHT	REST	SETS	REPS	WEIGHT	REST	SETS	REPS	WEIGHT	REST	SETS	REPS	WEIGHT	REST

CARDIO:	TIME	DIST.	INT.	PACE	TIME	DIST.	INT.	PACE	TIME	DIST.	INT.	PACE	TIME	DIST.	INT.	PACE

WORKOUT LOG

NAME:
GOALS:
DATE:
STATS:
WEIGHT:

EXERCISE:	SETS	REPS	WEIGHT	REST	SETS	REPS	WEIGHT	REST	SETS	REPS	WEIGHT	REST	SETS	REPS	WEIGHT	REST

CARDIO:	TIME	DIST.	INT.	PACE	TIME	DIST.	INT.	PACE	TIME	DIST.	INT.	PACE	TIME	DIST.	INT.	PACE

WORKOUT LOG

NAME:

GOALS:

DATE:

STATS:

WEIGHT:

EXERCISE:	SETS	REPS	WEIGHT	REST	SETS	REPS	WEIGHT	REST	SETS	REPS	WEIGHT	REST	SETS	REPS	WEIGHT	REST

CARDIO:	TIME	DIST.	INT.	PACE	TIME	DIST.	INT.	PACE	TIME	DIST.	INT.	PACE	TIME	DIST.	INT.	PACE

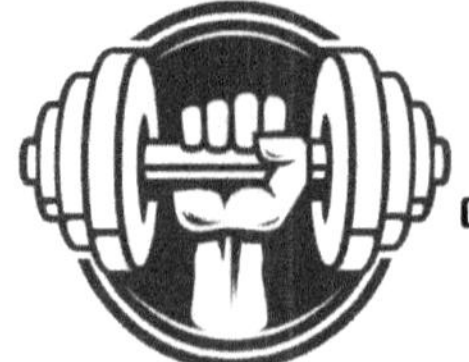

WORKOUT LOG

NAME:

GOALS:

DATE:

STATS:

WEIGHT:

EXERCISE:	SETS	REPS	WEIGHT	REST	SETS	REPS	WEIGHT	REST	SETS	REPS	WEIGHT	REST	SETS	REPS	WEIGHT	REST

CARDIO:	TIME	DIST.	INT.	PACE	TIME	DIST.	INT.	PACE	TIME	DIST.	INT.	PACE	TIME	DIST.	INT.	PACE

WORKOUT LOG

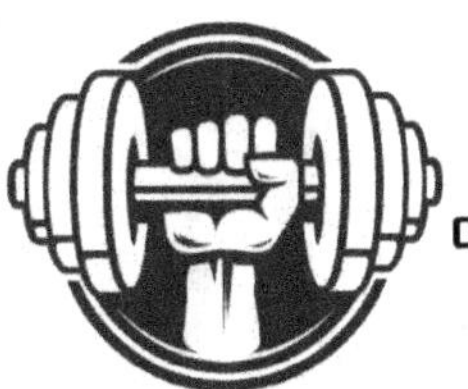

NAME:

GOALS:

DATE:

STATS:

WEIGHT:

EXERCISE:	SETS	REPS	WEIGHT	REST	SETS	REPS	WEIGHT	REST	SETS	REPS	WEIGHT	REST	SETS	REPS	WEIGHT	REST

CARDIO:	TIME	DIST.	INT.	PACE	TIME	DIST.	INT.	PACE	TIME	DIST.	INT.	PACE	TIME	DIST.	INT.	PACE

WORKOUT LOG

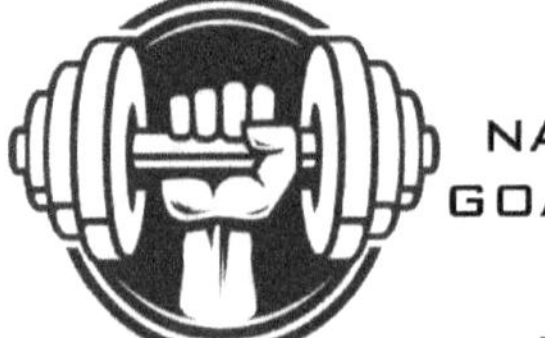

NAME:
GOALS:
DATE:
STATS:
WEIGHT:

EXERCISE:	SETS	REPS	WEIGHT	REST	SETS	REPS	WEIGHT	REST	SETS	REPS	WEIGHT	REST	SETS	REPS	WEIGHT	REST

CARDIO:	TIME	DIST.	INT.	PACE	TIME	DIST.	INT.	PACE	TIME	DIST.	INT.	PACE	TIME	DIST.	INT.	PACE

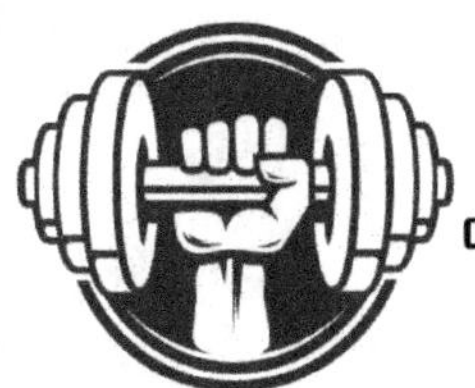

WORKOUT LOG

NAME:

GOALS:

DATE:

STATS:

WEIGHT:

EXERCISE:	SETS	REPS	WEIGHT	REST	SETS	REPS	WEIGHT	REST	SETS	REPS	WEIGHT	REST	SETS	REPS	WEIGHT	REST

CARDIO:	TIME	DIST.	INT.	PACE	TIME	DIST.	INT.	PACE	TIME	DIST.	INT.	PACE	TIME	DIST.	INT.	PACE

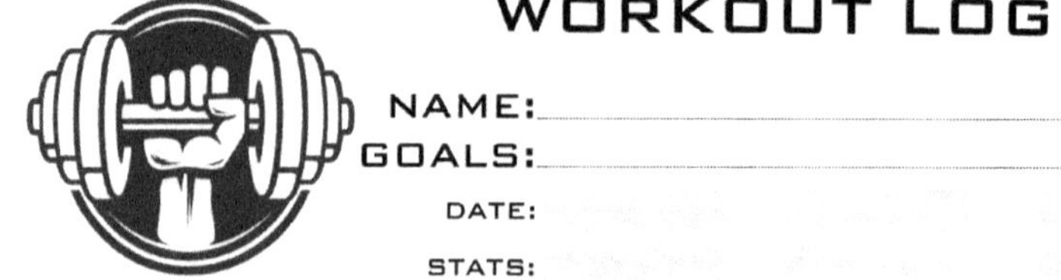

WORKOUT LOG

NAME:

GOALS:

DATE:

STATS:

WEIGHT:

EXERCISE:	SETS	REPS	WEIGHT	REST	SETS	REPS	WEIGHT	REST	SETS	REPS	WEIGHT	REST	SETS	REPS	WEIGHT	REST

CARDIO:	TIME	DIST.	INT.	PACE	TIME	DIST.	INT.	PACE	TIME	DIST.	INT.	PACE	TIME	DIST.	INT.	PACE

WORKOUT LOG

NAME: ________________________

GOALS: ________________________

DATE: ________________________

STATS: ________________________

WEIGHT: ________________________

EXERCISE:	SETS	REPS	WEIGHT	REST	SETS	REPS	WEIGHT	REST	SETS	REPS	WEIGHT	REST	SETS	REPS	WEIGHT	REST

CARDIO:	TIME	DIST.	INT.	PACE	TIME	DIST.	INT.	PACE	TIME	DIST.	INT.	PACE	TIME	DIST.	INT.	PACE

WORKOUT LOG

NAME:

GOALS:

DATE:

STATS:

WEIGHT:

EXERCISE:	SETS	REPS	WEIGHT	REST	SETS	REPS	WEIGHT	REST	SETS	REPS	WEIGHT	REST	SETS	REPS	WEIGHT	REST

CARDIO:	TIME	DIST.	INT.	PACE	TIME	DIST.	INT.	PACE	TIME	DIST.	INT.	PACE	TIME	DIST.	INT.	PACE

WORKOUT LOG

NAME:

GOALS:

DATE:

STATS:

WEIGHT:

EXERCISE:	SETS	REPS	WEIGHT	REST	SETS	REPS	WEIGHT	REST	SETS	REPS	WEIGHT	REST	SETS	REPS	WEIGHT	REST

CARDIO:	TIME	DIST.	INT.	PACE	TIME	DIST.	INT.	PACE	TIME	DIST.	INT.	PACE	TIME	DIST.	INT.	PACE

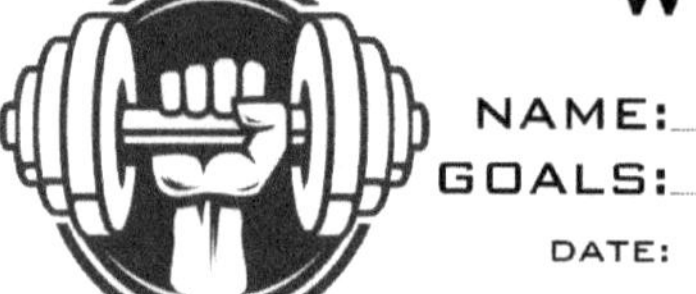

WORKOUT LOG

NAME:
GOALS:
DATE:
STATS:
WEIGHT:

EXERCISE:	SETS	REPS	WEIGHT	REST	SETS	REPS	WEIGHT	REST	SETS	REPS	WEIGHT	REST	SETS	REPS	WEIGHT	REST

CARDIO:	TIME	DIST.	INT.	PACE	TIME	DIST.	INT.	PACE	TIME	DIST.	INT.	PACE	TIME	DIST.	INT.	PACE

WORKOUT LOG

NAME:

GOALS:

DATE:

STATS:

WEIGHT:

EXERCISE:	SETS	REPS	WEIGHT	REST	SETS	REPS	WEIGHT	REST	SETS	REPS	WEIGHT	REST	SETS	REPS	WEIGHT	REST

CARDIO:	TIME	DIST.	INT.	PACE	TIME	DIST.	INT.	PACE	TIME	DIST.	INT.	PACE	TIME	DIST.	INT.	PACE

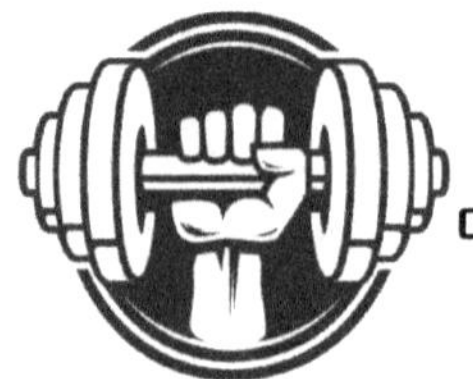

WORKOUT LOG

NAME:

GOALS:

DATE:

STATS:

WEIGHT:

EXERCISE:	SETS	REPS	WEIGHT	REST	SETS	REPS	WEIGHT	REST	SETS	REPS	WEIGHT	REST	SETS	REPS	WEIGHT	REST

CARDIO:	TIME	DIST.	INT.	PACE	TIME	DIST.	INT.	PACE	TIME	DIST.	INT.	PACE	TIME	DIST.	INT.	PACE

WORKOUT LOG

NAME:

GOALS:

DATE:

STATS:

WEIGHT:

EXERCISE:	SETS	REPS	WEIGHT	REST	SETS	REPS	WEIGHT	REST	SETS	REPS	WEIGHT	REST	SETS	REPS	WEIGHT	REST

CARDIO:	TIME	DIST.	INT.	PACE	TIME	DIST.	INT.	PACE	TIME	DIST.	INT.	PACE	TIME	DIST.	INT.	PACE

WORKOUT LOG

NAME:
GOALS:
DATE:
STATS:
WEIGHT:

EXERCISE:	SETS	REPS	WEIGHT	REST	SETS	REPS	WEIGHT	REST	SETS	REPS	WEIGHT	REST	SETS	REPS	WEIGHT	REST

CARDIO:	TIME	DIST.	INT.	PACE	TIME	DIST.	INT.	PACE	TIME	DIST.	INT.	PACE	TIME	DIST.	INT.	PACE

WORKOUT LOG

NAME: _______________________

GOALS: _______________________

DATE:

STATS:

WEIGHT:

EXERCISE:	SETS	REPS	WEIGHT	REST	SETS	REPS	WEIGHT	REST	SETS	REPS	WEIGHT	REST	SETS	REPS	WEIGHT	REST

CARDIO:	TIME	DIST.	INT.	PACE	TIME	DIST.	INT.	PACE	TIME	DIST.	INT.	PACE	TIME	DIST.	INT.	PACE

WORKOUT LOG

NAME:

GOALS:

DATE:

STATS:

WEIGHT:

EXERCISE:	SETS	REPS	WEIGHT	REST	SETS	REPS	WEIGHT	REST	SETS	REPS	WEIGHT	REST	SETS	REPS	WEIGHT	REST

CARDIO:	TIME	DIST.	INT.	PACE	TIME	DIST.	INT.	PACE	TIME	DIST.	INT.	PACE	TIME	DIST.	INT.	PACE

WORKOUT LOG

NAME:

GOALS:

DATE:

STATS:

WEIGHT:

EXERCISE:	SETS	REPS	WEIGHT	REST	SETS	REPS	WEIGHT	REST	SETS	REPS	WEIGHT	REST	SETS	REPS	WEIGHT	REST

CARDIO:	TIME	DIST.	INT.	PACE	TIME	DIST.	INT.	PACE	TIME	DIST.	INT.	PACE	TIME	DIST.	INT.	PACE

WORKOUT LOG

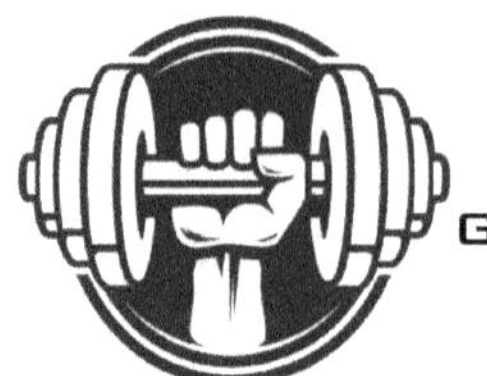

NAME:

GOALS:

DATE:

STATS:

WEIGHT:

EXERCISE:	SETS	REPS	WEIGHT	REST	SETS	REPS	WEIGHT	REST	SETS	REPS	WEIGHT	REST	SETS	REPS	WEIGHT	REST

CARDIO:	TIME	DIST.	INT.	PACE	TIME	DIST.	INT.	PACE	TIME	DIST.	INT.	PACE	TIME	DIST.	INT.	PACE

WORKOUT LOG

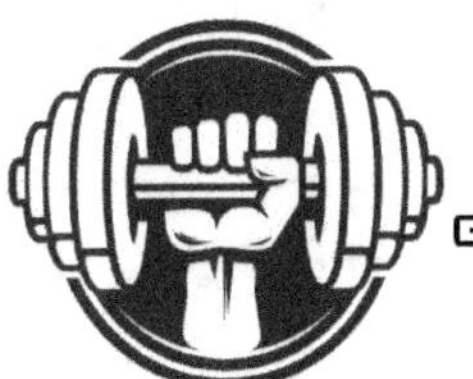

NAME:

GOALS:

DATE:

STATS:

WEIGHT:

EXERCISE:	SETS	REPS	WEIGHT	REST	SETS	REPS	WEIGHT	REST	SETS	REPS	WEIGHT	REST	SETS	REPS	WEIGHT	REST

CARDIO:	TIME	DIST.	INT.	PACE	TIME	DIST.	INT.	PACE	TIME	DIST.	INT.	PACE	TIME	DIST.	INT.	PACE

WORKOUT LOG

NAME:

GOALS:

DATE:

STATS:

WEIGHT:

EXERCISE:	SETS	REPS	WEIGHT	REST	SETS	REPS	WEIGHT	REST	SETS	REPS	WEIGHT	REST	SETS	REPS	WEIGHT	REST

CARDIO:	TIME	DIST.	INT.	PACE	TIME	DIST.	INT.	PACE	TIME	DIST.	INT.	PACE	TIME	DIST.	INT.	PACE

WORKOUT LOG

NAME: ___________________________

GOALS: ___________________________

DATE:

STATS:

WEIGHT:

EXERCISE:	SETS	REPS	WEIGHT	REST	SETS	REPS	WEIGHT	REST	SETS	REPS	WEIGHT	REST	SETS	REPS	WEIGHT	REST

CARDIO:	TIME	DIST.	INT.	PACE	TIME	DIST.	INT.	PACE	TIME	DIST.	INT.	PACE	TIME	DIST.	INT.	PACE

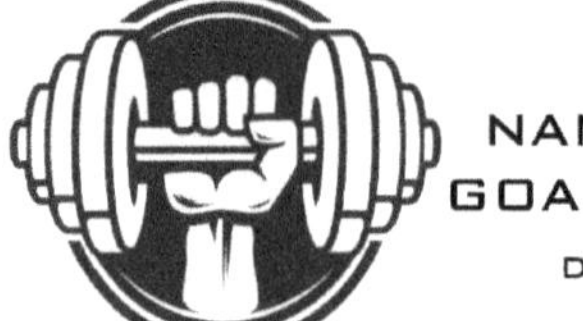

WORKOUT LOG

NAME:

GOALS:

DATE:

STATS:

WEIGHT:

EXERCISE:	SETS	REPS	WEIGHT	REST	SETS	REPS	WEIGHT	REST	SETS	REPS	WEIGHT	REST	SETS	REPS	WEIGHT	REST

CARDIO:	TIME	DIST.	INT.	PACE	TIME	DIST.	INT.	PACE	TIME	DIST.	INT.	PACE	TIME	DIST.	INT.	PACE

WORKOUT LOG

NAME: ___________________________

GOALS: ___________________________

DATE:

STATS:

WEIGHT:

EXERCISE:	SETS	REPS	WEIGHT	REST	SETS	REPS	WEIGHT	REST	SETS	REPS	WEIGHT	REST	SETS	REPS	WEIGHT	REST

CARDIO:	TIME	DIST.	INT.	PACE	TIME	DIST.	INT.	PACE	TIME	DIST.	INT.	PACE	TIME	DIST.	INT.	PACE

WORKOUT LOG

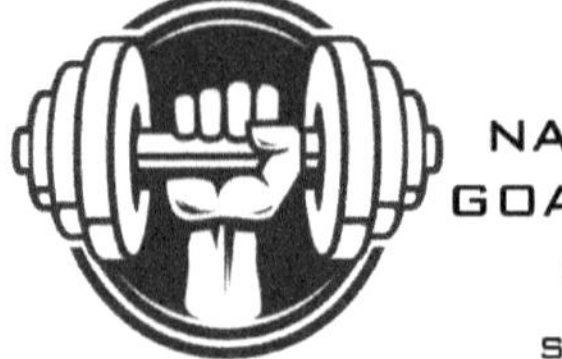

NAME:

GOALS:

DATE:

STATS:

WEIGHT:

EXERCISE:	SETS	REPS	WEIGHT	REST	SETS	REPS	WEIGHT	REST	SETS	REPS	WEIGHT	REST	SETS	REPS	WEIGHT	REST

CARDIO:	TIME	DIST.	INT.	PACE	TIME	DIST.	INT.	PACE	TIME	DIST.	INT.	PACE	TIME	DIST.	INT.	PACE

WORKOUT LOG

NAME:

GOALS:

DATE:

STATS:

WEIGHT:

EXERCISE:	SETS	REPS	WEIGHT	REST	SETS	REPS	WEIGHT	REST	SETS	REPS	WEIGHT	REST	SETS	REPS	WEIGHT	REST

CARDIO:	TIME	DIST.	INT.	PACE	TIME	DIST.	INT.	PACE	TIME	DIST.	INT.	PACE	TIME	DIST.	INT.	PACE

WORKOUT LOG

NAME:
GOALS:
DATE:
STATS:
WEIGHT:

EXERCISE:	SETS	REPS	WEIGHT	REST	SETS	REPS	WEIGHT	REST	SETS	REPS	WEIGHT	REST	SETS	REPS	WEIGHT	REST

CARDIO:	TIME	DIST.	INT.	PACE	TIME	DIST.	INT.	PACE	TIME	DIST.	INT.	PACE	TIME	DIST.	INT.	PACE

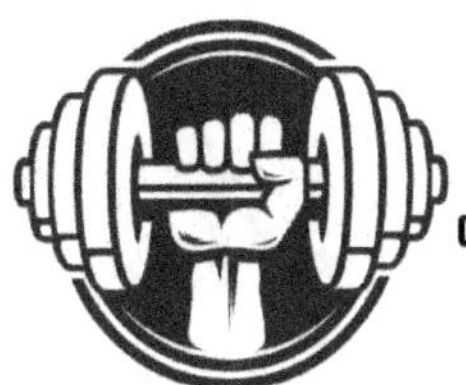

WORKOUT LOG

NAME:
GOALS:
DATE:
STATS:
WEIGHT:

EXERCISE:	SETS	REPS	WEIGHT	REST	SETS	REPS	WEIGHT	REST	SETS	REPS	WEIGHT	REST	SETS	REPS	WEIGHT	REST

CARDIO:	TIME	DIST.	INT.	PACE	TIME	DIST.	INT.	PACE	TIME	DIST.	INT.	PACE	TIME	DIST.	INT.	PACE

WORKOUT LOG

NAME:

GOALS:

DATE:

STATS:

WEIGHT:

EXERCISE:	SETS	REPS	WEIGHT	REST	SETS	REPS	WEIGHT	REST	SETS	REPS	WEIGHT	REST	SETS	REPS	WEIGHT	REST

CARDIO:	TIME	DIST.	INT.	PACE	TIME	DIST.	INT.	PACE	TIME	DIST.	INT.	PACE	TIME	DIST.	INT.	PACE

WORKOUT LOG

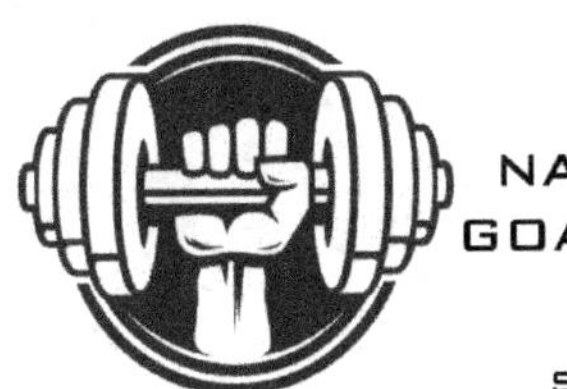

NAME:

GOALS:

DATE:

STATS:

WEIGHT:

EXERCISE:	SETS	REPS	WEIGHT	REST	SETS	REPS	WEIGHT	REST	SETS	REPS	WEIGHT	REST	SETS	REPS	WEIGHT	REST

CARDIO:	TIME	DIST.	INT.	PACE	TIME	DIST.	INT.	PACE	TIME	DIST.	INT.	PACE	TIME	DIST.	INT.	PACE

WORKOUT LOG

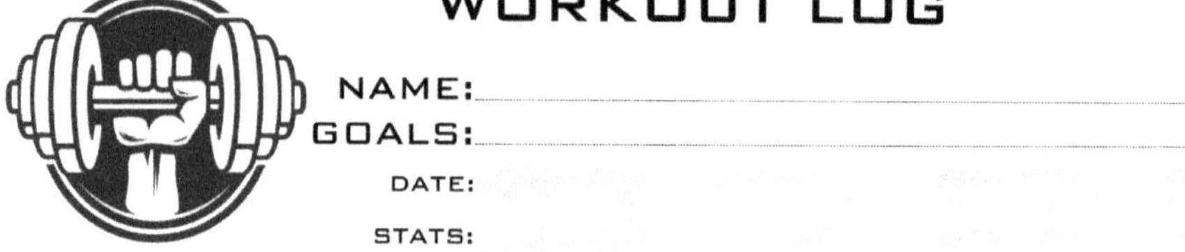

NAME:

GOALS:

DATE:

STATS:

WEIGHT:

EXERCISE:	SETS	REPS	WEIGHT	REST	SETS	REPS	WEIGHT	REST	SETS	REPS	WEIGHT	REST	SETS	REPS	WEIGHT	REST

CARDIO:	TIME	DIST.	INT.	PACE	TIME	DIST.	INT.	PACE	TIME	DIST.	INT.	PACE	TIME	DIST.	INT.	PACE

WORKOUT LOG

NAME:

GOALS:

DATE:

STATS:

WEIGHT:

EXERCISE:	SETS	REPS	WEIGHT	REST	SETS	REPS	WEIGHT	REST	SETS	REPS	WEIGHT	REST	SETS	REPS	WEIGHT	REST

CARDIO:	TIME	DIST.	INT.	PACE	TIME	DIST.	INT.	PACE	TIME	DIST.	INT.	PACE	TIME	DIST.	INT.	PACE

WORKOUT LOG

NAME:
GOALS:
DATE:
STATS:
WEIGHT:

EXERCISE:	SETS	REPS	WEIGHT	REST	SETS	REPS	WEIGHT	REST	SETS	REPS	WEIGHT	REST	SETS	REPS	WEIGHT	REST

CARDIO:	TIME	DIST.	INT.	PACE	TIME	DIST.	INT.	PACE	TIME	DIST.	INT.	PACE	TIME	DIST.	INT.	PACE

WORKOUT LOG

NAME:

GOALS:

DATE:

STATS:

WEIGHT:

EXERCISE:	SETS	REPS	WEIGHT	REST	SETS	REPS	WEIGHT	REST	SETS	REPS	WEIGHT	REST	SETS	REPS	WEIGHT	REST

CARDIO:	TIME	DIST.	INT.	PACE	TIME	DIST.	INT.	PACE	TIME	DIST.	INT.	PACE	TIME	DIST.	INT.	PACE

WORKOUT LOG

NAME:
GOALS:
DATE:
STATS:
WEIGHT:

EXERCISE:	SETS	REPS	WEIGHT	REST	SETS	REPS	WEIGHT	REST	SETS	REPS	WEIGHT	REST	SETS	REPS	WEIGHT	REST

CARDIO:	TIME	DIST.	INT.	PACE	TIME	DIST.	INT.	PACE	TIME	DIST.	INT.	PACE	TIME	DIST.	INT.	PACE

WORKOUT LOG

NAME: ___________________________
GOALS: ___________________________
DATE: ___________________________
STATS: ___________________________
WEIGHT: ___________________________

EXERCISE:	SETS	REPS	WEIGHT	REST	SETS	REPS	WEIGHT	REST	SETS	REPS	WEIGHT	REST	SETS	REPS	WEIGHT	REST

CARDIO:	TIME	DIST.	INT.	PACE	TIME	DIST.	INT.	PACE	TIME	DIST.	INT.	PACE	TIME	DIST.	INT.	PACE

WORKOUT LOG

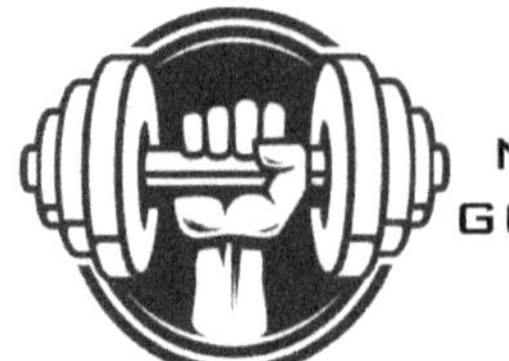

NAME:

GOALS:

DATE:

STATS:

WEIGHT:

EXERCISE:	SETS	REPS	WEIGHT	REST	SETS	REPS	WEIGHT	REST	SETS	REPS	WEIGHT	REST	SETS	REPS	WEIGHT	REST

CARDIO:	TIME	DIST.	INT.	PACE	TIME	DIST.	INT.	PACE	TIME	DIST.	INT.	PACE	TIME	DIST.	INT.	PACE

WORKOUT LOG

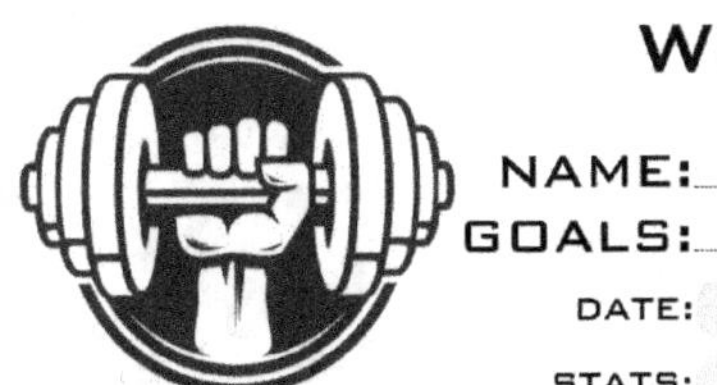

NAME: ___________________

GOALS: ___________________

DATE:

STATS:

WEIGHT:

EXERCISE:	SETS	REPS	WEIGHT	REST	SETS	REPS	WEIGHT	REST	SETS	REPS	WEIGHT	REST	SETS	REPS	WEIGHT	REST

CARDIO:	TIME	DIST.	INT.	PACE	TIME	DIST.	INT.	PACE	TIME	DIST.	INT.	PACE	TIME	DIST.	INT.	PACE

WORKOUT LOG

NAME: ....

GOALS: ....

DATE:

STATS:

WEIGHT:

EXERCISE:	SETS	REPS	WEIGHT	REST	SETS	REPS	WEIGHT	REST	SETS	REPS	WEIGHT	REST	SETS	REPS	WEIGHT	REST

CARDIO:	TIME	DIST.	INT.	PACE	TIME	DIST.	INT.	PACE	TIME	DIST.	INT.	PACE	TIME	DIST.	INT.	PACE

WORKOUT LOG

NAME:

GOALS:

DATE:

STATS:

WEIGHT:

EXERCISE:	SETS	REPS	WEIGHT	REST	SETS	REPS	WEIGHT	REST	SETS	REPS	WEIGHT	REST	SETS	REPS	WEIGHT	REST

CARDIO:	TIME	DIST.	INT.	PACE	TIME	DIST.	INT.	PACE	TIME	DIST.	INT.	PACE	TIME	DIST.	INT.	PACE

WORKOUT LOG

NAME:
GOALS:
DATE:
STATS:
WEIGHT:

EXERCISE:	SETS	REPS	WEIGHT	REST	SETS	REPS	WEIGHT	REST	SETS	REPS	WEIGHT	REST	SETS	REPS	WEIGHT	REST

CARDIO:	TIME	DIST.	INT.	PACE	TIME	DIST.	INT.	PACE	TIME	DIST.	INT.	PACE	TIME	DIST.	INT.	PACE

WORKOUT LOG

NAME:
GOALS:
DATE:
STATS:
WEIGHT:

EXERCISE:	SETS	REPS	WEIGHT	REST	SETS	REPS	WEIGHT	REST	SETS	REPS	WEIGHT	REST	SETS	REPS	WEIGHT	REST

CARDIO:	TIME	DIST.	INT.	PACE	TIME	DIST.	INT.	PACE	TIME	DIST.	INT.	PACE	TIME	DIST.	INT.	PACE

WORKOUT LOG

NAME:

GOALS:

DATE:

STATS:

WEIGHT:

EXERCISE:	SETS	REPS	WEIGHT	REST	SETS	REPS	WEIGHT	REST	SETS	REPS	WEIGHT	REST	SETS	REPS	WEIGHT	REST

CARDIO:	TIME	DIST.	INT.	PACE	TIME	DIST.	INT.	PACE	TIME	DIST.	INT.	PACE	TIME	DIST.	INT.	PACE

WORKOUT LOG

NAME:
GOALS:
DATE:
STATS:
WEIGHT:

EXERCISE:	SETS	REPS	WEIGHT	REST	SETS	REPS	WEIGHT	REST	SETS	REPS	WEIGHT	REST	SETS	REPS	WEIGHT	REST

CARDIO:	TIME	DIST.	INT.	PACE	TIME	DIST.	INT.	PACE	TIME	DIST.	INT.	PACE	TIME	DIST.	INT.	PACE

WORKOUT LOG

NAME:
GOALS:
DATE:
STATS:
WEIGHT:

EXERCISE:	SETS	REPS	WEIGHT	REST	SETS	REPS	WEIGHT	REST	SETS	REPS	WEIGHT	REST	SETS	REPS	WEIGHT	REST

CARDIO:	TIME	DIST.	INT.	PACE	TIME	DIST.	INT.	PACE	TIME	DIST.	INT.	PACE	TIME	DIST.	INT.	PACE

WORKOUT LOG

NAME: ______________________

GOALS: ______________________

DATE:

STATS:

WEIGHT:

EXERCISE:	SETS	REPS	WEIGHT	REST	SETS	REPS	WEIGHT	REST	SETS	REPS	WEIGHT	REST	SETS	REPS	WEIGHT	REST

CARDIO:	TIME	DIST.	INT.	PACE	TIME	DIST.	INT.	PACE	TIME	DIST.	INT.	PACE	TIME	DIST.	INT.	PACE

WORKOUT LOG

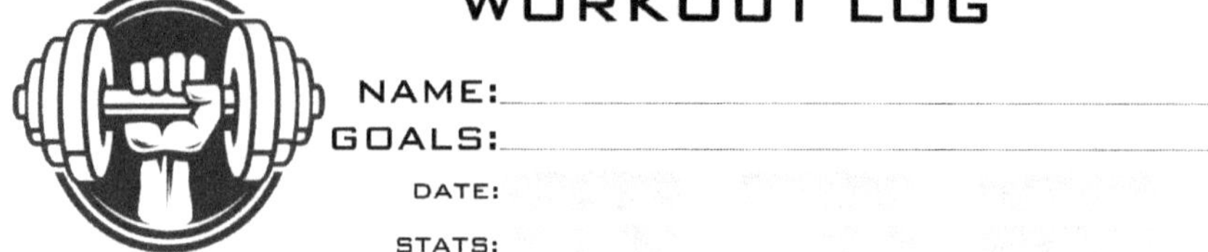

NAME:

GOALS:

DATE:

STATS:

WEIGHT:

EXERCISE:	SETS	REPS	WEIGHT	REST	SETS	REPS	WEIGHT	REST	SETS	REPS	WEIGHT	REST	SETS	REPS	WEIGHT	REST

CARDIO:	TIME	DIST.	INT.	PACE	TIME	DIST.	INT.	PACE	TIME	DIST.	INT.	PACE	TIME	DIST.	INT.	PACE

WORKOUT LOG

NAME:
GOALS:
DATE:
STATS:
WEIGHT:

EXERCISE:	SETS	REPS	WEIGHT	REST	SETS	REPS	WEIGHT	REST	SETS	REPS	WEIGHT	REST	SETS	REPS	WEIGHT	REST

CARDIO:	TIME	DIST.	INT.	PACE	TIME	DIST.	INT.	PACE	TIME	DIST.	INT.	PACE	TIME	DIST.	INT.	PACE

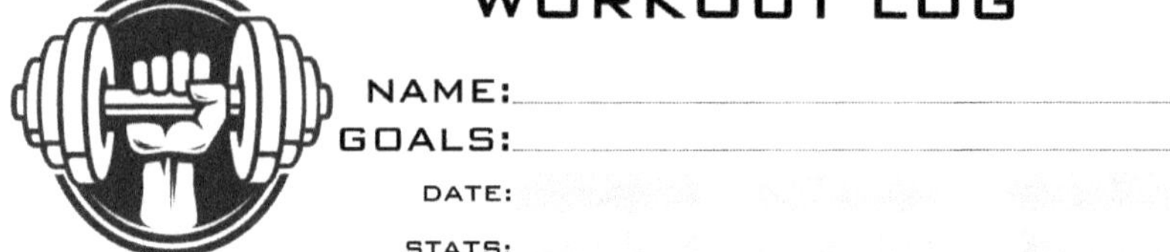

WORKOUT LOG

NAME:
GOALS:
DATE:
STATS:
WEIGHT:

EXERCISE:	SETS	REPS	WEIGHT	REST	SETS	REPS	WEIGHT	REST	SETS	REPS	WEIGHT	REST	SETS	REPS	WEIGHT	REST

CARDIO:	TIME	DIST.	INT.	PACE	TIME	DIST.	INT.	PACE	TIME	DIST.	INT.	PACE	TIME	DIST.	INT.	PACE

WORKOUT LOG

NAME:
GOALS:
DATE:
STATS:
WEIGHT:

EXERCISE:	SETS	REPS	WEIGHT	REST	SETS	REPS	WEIGHT	REST	SETS	REPS	WEIGHT	REST	SETS	REPS	WEIGHT	REST

CARDIO:	TIME	DIST.	INT.	PACE	TIME	DIST.	INT.	PACE	TIME	DIST.	INT.	PACE	TIME	DIST.	INT.	PACE

WORKOUT LOG

NAME:
GOALS:
DATE:
STATS:
WEIGHT:

EXERCISE:	SETS	REPS	WEIGHT	REST	SETS	REPS	WEIGHT	REST	SETS	REPS	WEIGHT	REST	SETS	REPS	WEIGHT	REST

CARDIO:	TIME	DIST.	INT.	PACE	TIME	DIST.	INT.	PACE	TIME	DIST.	INT.	PACE	TIME	DIST.	INT.	PACE

WORKOUT LOG

NAME:
GOALS:
DATE:
STATS:
WEIGHT:

EXERCISE:	SETS	REPS	WEIGHT	REST	SETS	REPS	WEIGHT	REST	SETS	REPS	WEIGHT	REST	SETS	REPS	WEIGHT	REST

CARDIO:	TIME	DIST.	INT.	PACE	TIME	DIST.	INT.	PACE	TIME	DIST.	INT.	PACE	TIME	DIST.	INT.	PACE

WORKOUT LOG

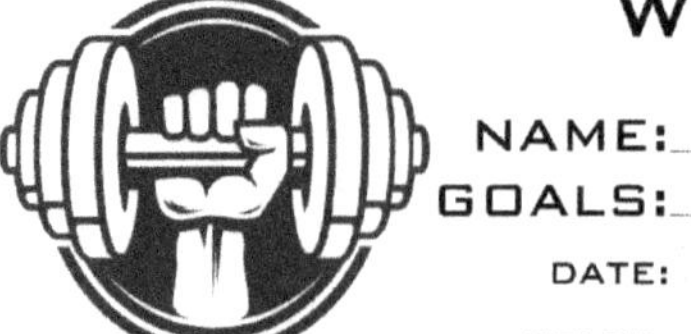

NAME:
GOALS:
DATE:
STATS:
WEIGHT:

EXERCISE:	SETS	REPS	WEIGHT	REST	SETS	REPS	WEIGHT	REST	SETS	REPS	WEIGHT	REST	SETS	REPS	WEIGHT	REST

CARDIO:	TIME	DIST.	INT.	PACE	TIME	DIST.	INT.	PACE	TIME	DIST.	INT.	PACE	TIME	DIST.	INT.	PACE

WORKOUT LOG

NAME:

GOALS:

DATE:

STATS:

WEIGHT:

EXERCISE:

	SETS	REPS	WEIGHT	REST	SETS	REPS	WEIGHT	REST	SETS	REPS	WEIGHT	REST	SETS	REPS	WEIGHT	REST

CARDIO:

	TIME	DIST.	INT.	PACE	TIME	DIST.	INT.	PACE	TIME	DIST.	INT.	PACE	TIME	DIST.	INT.	PACE

WORKOUT LOG

NAME:

GOALS:

DATE:

STATS:

WEIGHT:

EXERCISE:	SETS	REPS	WEIGHT	REST	SETS	REPS	WEIGHT	REST	SETS	REPS	WEIGHT	REST	SETS	REPS	WEIGHT	REST

CARDIO:	TIME	DIST.	INT.	PACE	TIME	DIST.	INT.	PACE	TIME	DIST.	INT.	PACE	TIME	DIST.	INT.	PACE

WORKOUT LOG

NAME:

GOALS:

DATE:

STATS:

WEIGHT:

EXERCISE:	SETS	REPS	WEIGHT	REST	SETS	REPS	WEIGHT	REST	SETS	REPS	WEIGHT	REST	SETS	REPS	WEIGHT	REST

CARDIO:	TIME	DIST.	INT.	PACE	TIME	DIST.	INT.	PACE	TIME	DIST.	INT.	PACE	TIME	DIST.	INT.	PACE

WORKOUT LOG

NAME: ____

GOALS: ____

DATE:

STATS:

WEIGHT:

EXERCISE:	SETS	REPS	WEIGHT	REST	SETS	REPS	WEIGHT	REST	SETS	REPS	WEIGHT	REST	SETS	REPS	WEIGHT	REST

CARDIO:	TIME	DIST.	INT.	PACE	TIME	DIST.	INT.	PACE	TIME	DIST.	INT.	PACE	TIME	DIST.	INT.	PACE

WORKOUT LOG

NAME:

GOALS:

DATE:

STATS:

WEIGHT:

EXERCISE:	SETS	REPS	WEIGHT	REST	SETS	REPS	WEIGHT	REST	SETS	REPS	WEIGHT	REST	SETS	REPS	WEIGHT	REST

CARDIO:	TIME	DIST.	INT.	PACE	TIME	DIST.	INT.	PACE	TIME	DIST.	INT.	PACE	TIME	DIST.	INT.	PACE

WORKOUT LOG

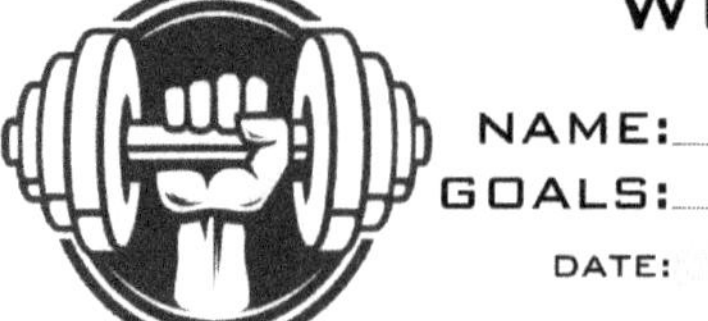

NAME:

GOALS:

DATE:

STATS:

WEIGHT:

EXERCISE:	SETS	REPS	WEIGHT	REST	SETS	REPS	WEIGHT	REST	SETS	REPS	WEIGHT	REST	SETS	REPS	WEIGHT	REST

CARDIO:	TIME	DIST.	INT.	PACE	TIME	DIST.	INT.	PACE	TIME	DIST.	INT.	PACE	TIME	DIST.	INT.	PACE

WORKOUT LOG

NAME:

GOALS:

DATE:

STATS:

WEIGHT:

EXERCISE:	SETS	REPS	WEIGHT	REST	SETS	REPS	WEIGHT	REST	SETS	REPS	WEIGHT	REST	SETS	REPS	WEIGHT	REST

CARDIO:	TIME	DIST.	INT.	PACE	TIME	DIST.	INT.	PACE	TIME	DIST.	INT.	PACE	TIME	DIST.	INT.	PACE

WORKOUT LOG

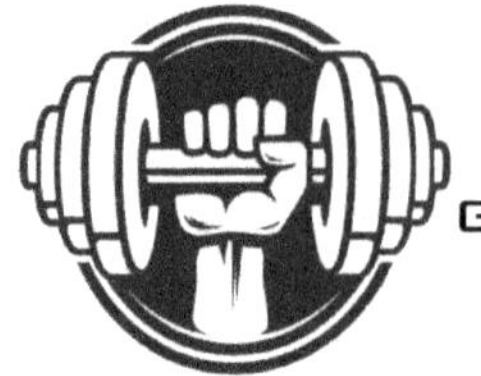

NAME:

GOALS:

DATE:

STATS:

WEIGHT:

EXERCISE:	SETS	REPS	WEIGHT	REST	SETS	REPS	WEIGHT	REST	SETS	REPS	WEIGHT	REST	SETS	REPS	WEIGHT	REST

CARDIO:	TIME	DIST.	INT.	PACE	TIME	DIST.	INT.	PACE	TIME	DIST.	INT.	PACE	TIME	DIST.	INT.	PACE

WORKOUT LOG

NAME:

GOALS:

DATE:

STATS:

WEIGHT:

EXERCISE:	SETS	REPS	WEIGHT	REST	SETS	REPS	WEIGHT	REST	SETS	REPS	WEIGHT	REST	SETS	REPS	WEIGHT	REST

CARDIO:	TIME	DIST.	INT.	PACE	TIME	DIST.	INT.	PACE	TIME	DIST.	INT.	PACE	TIME	DIST.	INT.	PACE

WORKOUT LOG

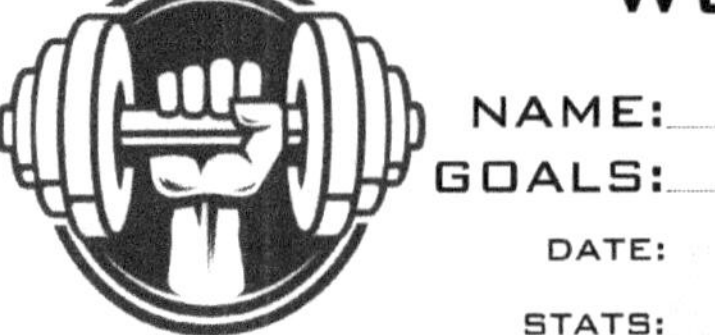

NAME:

GOALS:

DATE:

STATS:

WEIGHT:

EXERCISE:	SETS	REPS	WEIGHT	REST	SETS	REPS	WEIGHT	REST	SETS	REPS	WEIGHT	REST	SETS	REPS	WEIGHT	REST

CARDIO:	TIME	DIST.	INT.	PACE	TIME	DIST.	INT.	PACE	TIME	DIST.	INT.	PACE	TIME	DIST.	INT.	PACE

WORKOUT LOG

NAME:

GOALS:

DATE:

STATS:

WEIGHT:

EXERCISE:	SETS	REPS	WEIGHT	REST	SETS	REPS	WEIGHT	REST	SETS	REPS	WEIGHT	REST	SETS	REPS	WEIGHT	REST

CARDIO:	TIME	DIST.	INT.	PACE	TIME	DIST.	INT.	PACE	TIME	DIST.	INT.	PACE	TIME	DIST.	INT.	PACE

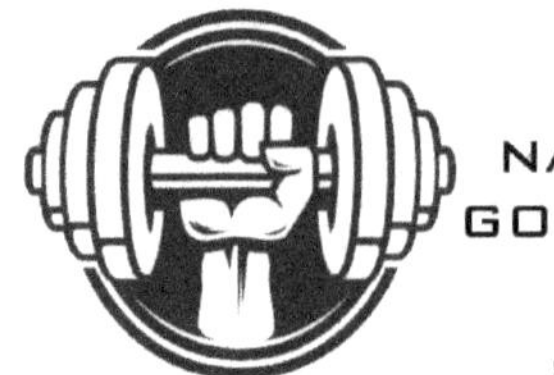

WORKOUT LOG

NAME:
GOALS:
DATE:
STATS:
WEIGHT:

EXERCISE:	SETS	REPS	WEIGHT	REST	SETS	REPS	WEIGHT	REST	SETS	REPS	WEIGHT	REST	SETS	REPS	WEIGHT	REST

CARDIO:	TIME	DIST.	INT.	PACE	TIME	DIST.	INT.	PACE	TIME	DIST.	INT.	PACE	TIME	DIST.	INT.	PACE

WORKOUT LOG

NAME:
GOALS:
DATE:
STATS:
WEIGHT:

EXERCISE:	SETS	REPS	WEIGHT	REST	SETS	REPS	WEIGHT	REST	SETS	REPS	WEIGHT	REST	SETS	REPS	WEIGHT	REST

CARDIO:	TIME	DIST.	INT.	PACE	TIME	DIST.	INT.	PACE	TIME	DIST.	INT.	PACE	TIME	DIST.	INT.	PACE

WORKOUT LOG

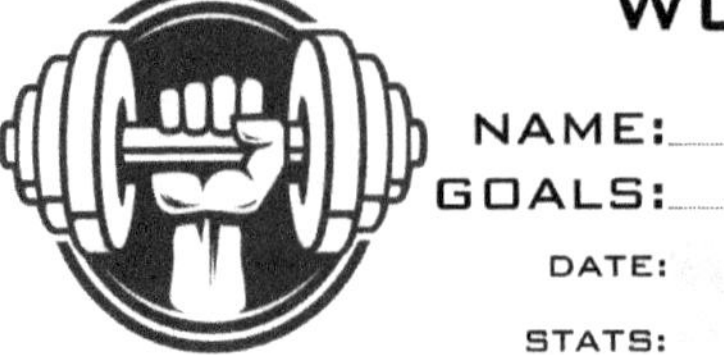

NAME:

GOALS:

DATE:

STATS:

WEIGHT:

EXERCISE:	SETS	REPS	WEIGHT	REST	SETS	REPS	WEIGHT	REST	SETS	REPS	WEIGHT	REST	SETS	REPS	WEIGHT	REST

CARDIO:	TIME	DIST.	INT.	PACE	TIME	DIST.	INT.	PACE	TIME	DIST.	INT.	PACE	TIME	DIST.	INT.	PACE

WORKOUT LOG

NAME: ________________________

GOALS: ________________________

DATE:

STATS:

WEIGHT:

EXERCISE:	SETS	REPS	WEIGHT	REST	SETS	REPS	WEIGHT	REST	SETS	REPS	WEIGHT	REST	SETS	REPS	WEIGHT	REST

CARDIO:	TIME	DIST.	INT.	PACE	TIME	DIST.	INT.	PACE	TIME	DIST.	INT.	PACE	TIME	DIST.	INT.	PACE

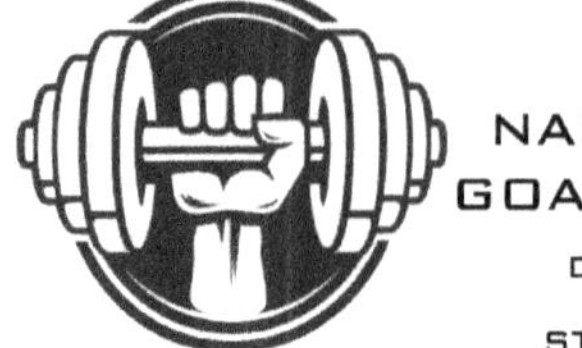

WORKOUT LOG

NAME:
GOALS:
DATE:
STATS:
WEIGHT:

EXERCISE:	SETS	REPS	WEIGHT	REST	SETS	REPS	WEIGHT	REST	SETS	REPS	WEIGHT	REST	SETS	REPS	WEIGHT	REST

CARDIO:	TIME	DIST.	INT.	PACE	TIME	DIST.	INT.	PACE	TIME	DIST.	INT.	PACE	TIME	DIST.	INT.	PACE

WORKOUT LOG

NAME:
GOALS:
DATE:
STATS:
WEIGHT:

EXERCISE:	SETS	REPS	WEIGHT	REST	SETS	REPS	WEIGHT	REST	SETS	REPS	WEIGHT	REST	SETS	REPS	WEIGHT	REST

CARDIO:	TIME	DIST.	INT.	PACE	TIME	DIST.	INT.	PACE	TIME	DIST.	INT.	PACE	TIME	DIST.	INT.	PACE

WORKOUT LOG

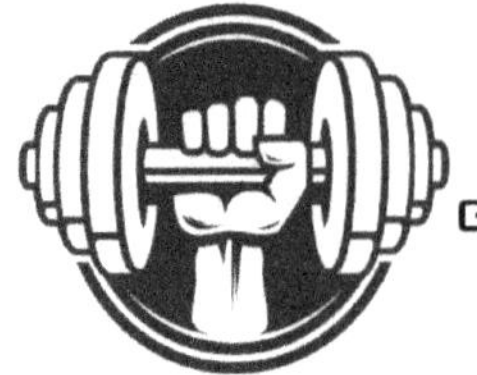

NAME:
GOALS:
DATE:
STATS:
WEIGHT:

EXERCISE:	SETS	REPS	WEIGHT	REST	SETS	REPS	WEIGHT	REST	SETS	REPS	WEIGHT	REST	SETS	REPS	WEIGHT	REST

CARDIO:	TIME	DIST.	INT.	PACE	TIME	DIST.	INT.	PACE	TIME	DIST.	INT.	PACE	TIME	DIST.	INT.	PACE

WORKOUT LOG

NAME:
GOALS:
DATE:
STATS:
WEIGHT:

EXERCISE:	SETS	REPS	WEIGHT	REST	SETS	REPS	WEIGHT	REST	SETS	REPS	WEIGHT	REST	SETS	REPS	WEIGHT	REST

CARDIO:	TIME	DIST.	INT.	PACE	TIME	DIST.	INT.	PACE	TIME	DIST.	INT.	PACE	TIME	DIST.	INT.	PACE

WORKOUT LOG

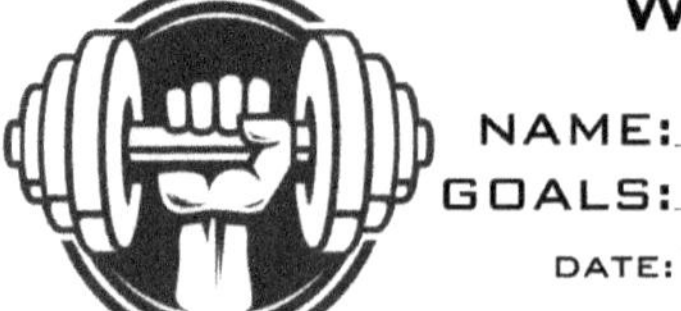

NAME:
GOALS:
DATE:
STATS:
WEIGHT:

EXERCISE:	SETS	REPS	WEIGHT	REST	SETS	REPS	WEIGHT	REST	SETS	REPS	WEIGHT	REST	SETS	REPS	WEIGHT	REST

CARDIO:	TIME	DIST.	INT.	PACE	TIME	DIST.	INT.	PACE	TIME	DIST.	INT.	PACE	TIME	DIST.	INT.	PACE

WORKOUT LOG

NAME:
GOALS:
DATE:
STATS:
WEIGHT:

EXERCISE:	SETS	REPS	WEIGHT	REST	SETS	REPS	WEIGHT	REST	SETS	REPS	WEIGHT	REST	SETS	REPS	WEIGHT	REST

CARDIO:	TIME	DIST.	INT.	PACE	TIME	DIST.	INT.	PACE	TIME	DIST.	INT.	PACE	TIME	DIST.	INT.	PACE

WORKOUT LOG

NAME:

GOALS:

DATE:

STATS:

WEIGHT:

EXERCISE:	SETS	REPS	WEIGHT	REST	SETS	REPS	WEIGHT	REST	SETS	REPS	WEIGHT	REST	SETS	REPS	WEIGHT	REST

CARDIO:	TIME	DIST.	INT.	PACE	TIME	DIST.	INT.	PACE	TIME	DIST.	INT.	PACE	TIME	DIST.	INT.	PACE

WORKOUT LOG

NAME:
GOALS:
DATE:
STATS:
WEIGHT:

EXERCISE:	SETS	REPS	WEIGHT	REST	SETS	REPS	WEIGHT	REST	SETS	REPS	WEIGHT	REST	SETS	REPS	WEIGHT	REST

CARDIO:	TIME	DIST.	INT.	PACE	TIME	DIST.	INT.	PACE	TIME	DIST.	INT.	PACE	TIME	DIST.	INT.	PACE

WORKOUT LOG

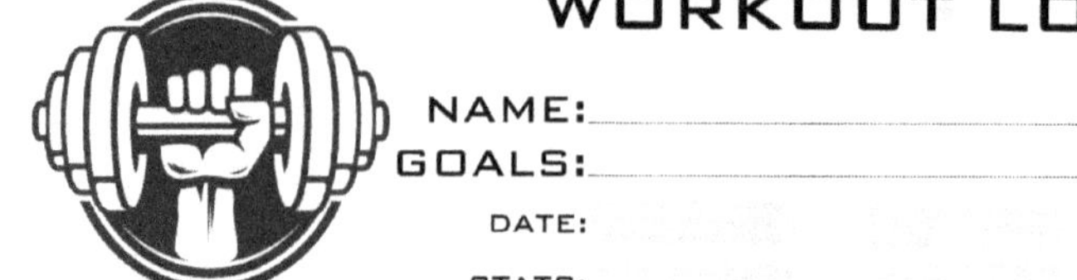

NAME:

GOALS:

DATE:

STATS:

WEIGHT:

EXERCISE:	SETS	REPS	WEIGHT	REST	SETS	REPS	WEIGHT	REST	SETS	REPS	WEIGHT	REST	SETS	REPS	WEIGHT	REST

CARDIO:	TIME	DIST.	INT.	PACE	TIME	DIST.	INT.	PACE	TIME	DIST.	INT.	PACE	TIME	DIST.	INT.	PACE

WORKOUT LOG

NAME:

GOALS:

DATE:

STATS:

WEIGHT:

EXERCISE:	SETS	REPS	WEIGHT	REST	SETS	REPS	WEIGHT	REST	SETS	REPS	WEIGHT	REST	SETS	REPS	WEIGHT	REST

CARDIO:	TIME	DIST.	INT.	PACE	TIME	DIST.	INT.	PACE	TIME	DIST.	INT.	PACE	TIME	DIST.	INT.	PACE

WORKOUT LOG

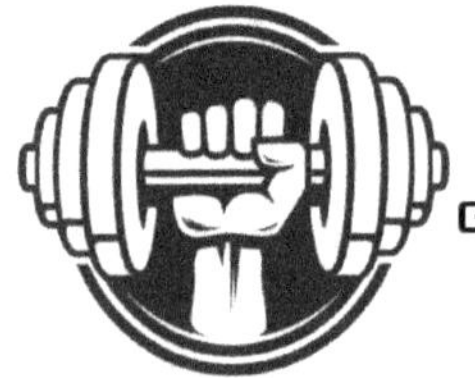

NAME:

GOALS:

DATE:

STATS:

WEIGHT:

EXERCISE:	SETS	REPS	WEIGHT	REST	SETS	REPS	WEIGHT	REST	SETS	REPS	WEIGHT	REST	SETS	REPS	WEIGHT	REST

CARDIO:	TIME	DIST.	INT.	PACE	TIME	DIST.	INT.	PACE	TIME	DIST.	INT.	PACE	TIME	DIST.	INT.	PACE

WORKOUT LOG

NAME:
GOALS:
DATE:
STATS:
WEIGHT:

EXERCISE:	SETS	REPS	WEIGHT	REST	SETS	REPS	WEIGHT	REST	SETS	REPS	WEIGHT	REST	SETS	REPS	WEIGHT	REST

CARDIO:	TIME	DIST.	INT.	PACE	TIME	DIST.	INT.	PACE	TIME	DIST.	INT.	PACE	TIME	DIST.	INT.	PACE

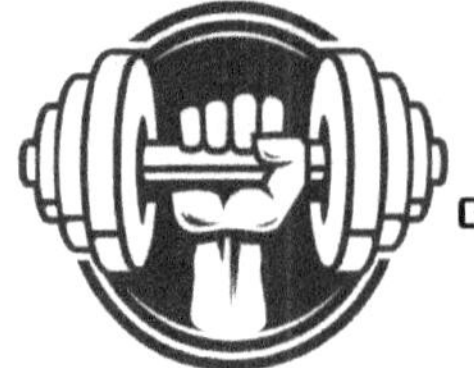

WORKOUT LOG

NAME:
GOALS:
DATE:
STATS:
WEIGHT:

EXERCISE:	SETS	REPS	WEIGHT	REST	SETS	REPS	WEIGHT	REST	SETS	REPS	WEIGHT	REST	SETS	REPS	WEIGHT	REST

CARDIO:	TIME	DIST.	INT.	PACE	TIME	DIST.	INT.	PACE	TIME	DIST.	INT.	PACE	TIME	DIST.	INT.	PACE

WORKOUT LOG

NAME:

GOALS:

DATE:

STATS:

WEIGHT:

EXERCISE:	SETS	REPS	WEIGHT	REST	SETS	REPS	WEIGHT	REST	SETS	REPS	WEIGHT	REST	SETS	REPS	WEIGHT	REST

CARDIO:	TIME	DIST.	INT.	PACE	TIME	DIST.	INT.	PACE	TIME	DIST.	INT.	PACE	TIME	DIST.	INT.	PACE

WORKOUT LOG

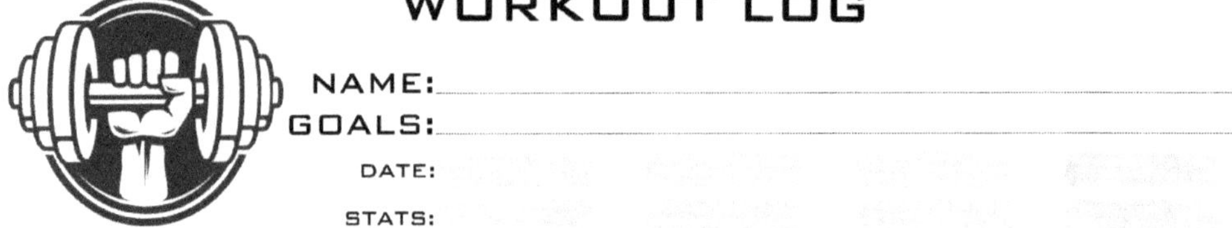

NAME:

GOALS:

DATE:

STATS:

WEIGHT:

EXERCISE:	SETS	REPS	WEIGHT	REST	SETS	REPS	WEIGHT	REST	SETS	REPS	WEIGHT	REST	SETS	REPS	WEIGHT	REST

CARDIO:	TIME	DIST.	INT.	PACE	TIME	DIST.	INT.	PACE	TIME	DIST.	INT.	PACE	TIME	DIST.	INT.	PACE

WORKOUT LOG

NAME:
GOALS:
DATE:
STATS:
WEIGHT:

EXERCISE:	SETS	REPS	WEIGHT	REST	SETS	REPS	WEIGHT	REST	SETS	REPS	WEIGHT	REST	SETS	REPS	WEIGHT	REST

CARDIO:	TIME	DIST.	INT.	PACE	TIME	DIST.	INT.	PACE	TIME	DIST.	INT.	PACE	TIME	DIST.	INT.	PACE

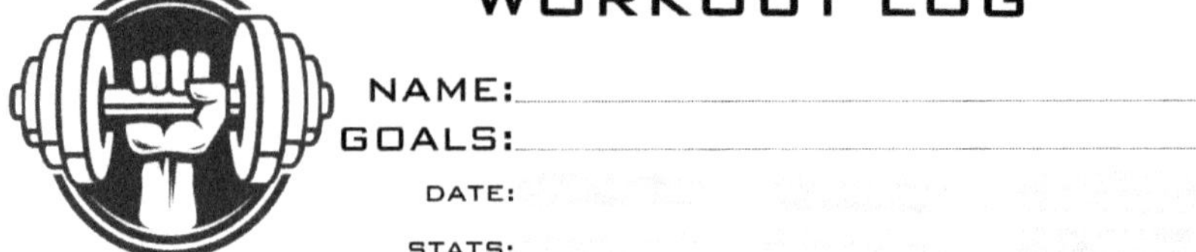

WORKOUT LOG

NAME:

GOALS:

DATE:

STATS:

WEIGHT:

EXERCISE:	SETS	REPS	WEIGHT	REST	SETS	REPS	WEIGHT	REST	SETS	REPS	WEIGHT	REST	SETS	REPS	WEIGHT	REST

CARDIO:	TIME	DIST.	INT.	PACE	TIME	DIST.	INT.	PACE	TIME	DIST.	INT.	PACE	TIME	DIST.	INT.	PACE

WORKOUT LOG

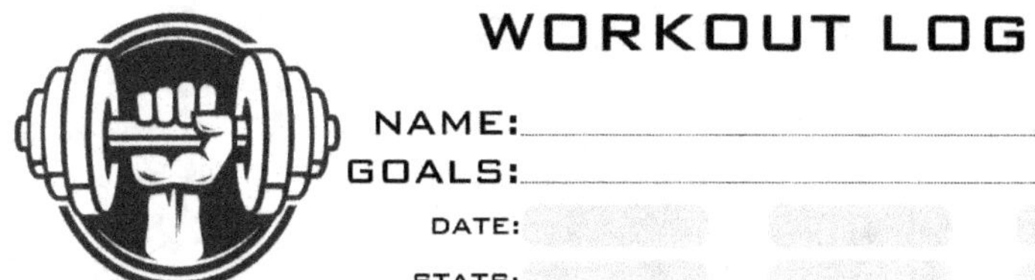

NAME:

GOALS:

DATE:

STATS:

WEIGHT:

EXERCISE:	SETS	REPS	WEIGHT	REST	SETS	REPS	WEIGHT	REST	SETS	REPS	WEIGHT	REST	SETS	REPS	WEIGHT	REST

CARDIO:	TIME	DIST.	INT.	PACE	TIME	DIST.	INT.	PACE	TIME	DIST.	INT.	PACE	TIME	DIST.	INT.	PACE

WORKOUT LOG

NAME:
GOALS:
DATE:
STATS:
WEIGHT:

EXERCISE:	SETS	REPS	WEIGHT	REST	SETS	REPS	WEIGHT	REST	SETS	REPS	WEIGHT	REST	SETS	REPS	WEIGHT	REST

CARDIO:	TIME	DIST.	INT.	PACE	TIME	DIST.	INT.	PACE	TIME	DIST.	INT.	PACE	TIME	DIST.	INT.	PACE

WORKOUT LOG

NAME:

GOALS:

DATE:

STATS:

WEIGHT:

EXERCISE:	SETS	REPS	WEIGHT	REST	SETS	REPS	WEIGHT	REST	SETS	REPS	WEIGHT	REST	SETS	REPS	WEIGHT	REST

CARDIO:	TIME	DIST.	INT.	PACE	TIME	DIST.	INT.	PACE	TIME	DIST.	INT.	PACE	TIME	DIST.	INT.	PACE

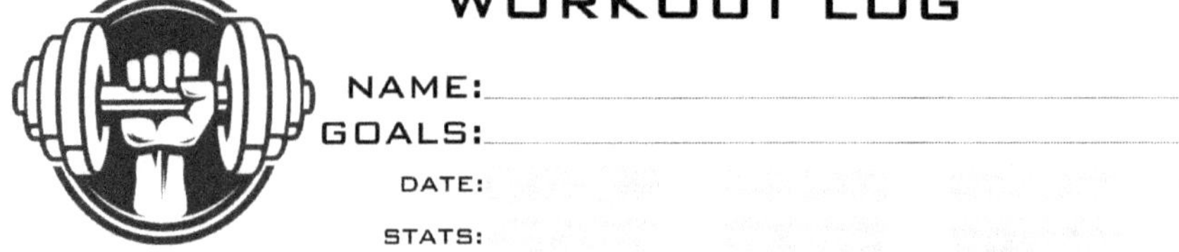

WORKOUT LOG

NAME:
GOALS:
DATE:
STATS:
WEIGHT:

EXERCISE:	SETS	REPS	WEIGHT	REST	SETS	REPS	WEIGHT	REST	SETS	REPS	WEIGHT	REST	SETS	REPS	WEIGHT	REST

CARDIO:	TIME	DIST.	INT.	PACE	TIME	DIST.	INT.	PACE	TIME	DIST.	INT.	PACE	TIME	DIST.	INT.	PACE

WORKOUT LOG

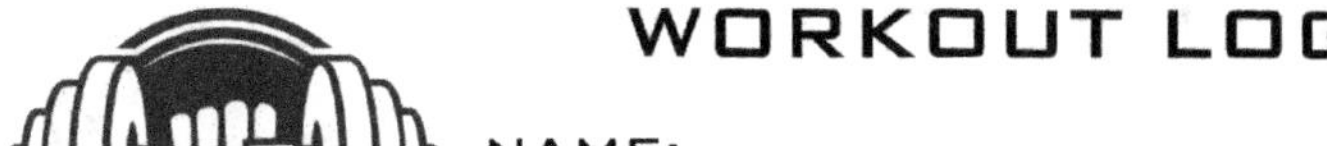

NAME:

GOALS:

DATE:

STATS:

WEIGHT:

EXERCISE:	SETS	REPS	WEIGHT	REST	SETS	REPS	WEIGHT	REST	SETS	REPS	WEIGHT	REST	SETS	REPS	WEIGHT	REST

CARDIO:	TIME	DIST.	INT.	PACE	TIME	DIST.	INT.	PACE	TIME	DIST.	INT.	PACE	TIME	DIST.	INT.	PACE

WORKOUT LOG

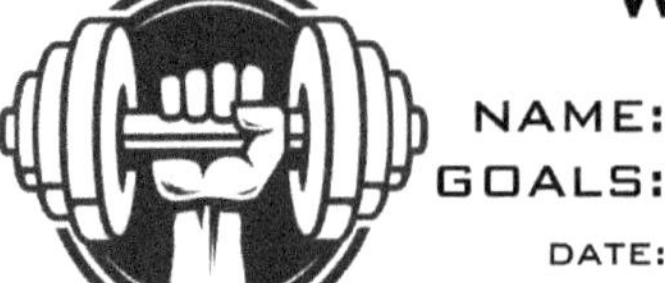

NAME:

GOALS:

DATE:

STATS:

WEIGHT:

EXERCISE:	SETS	REPS	WEIGHT	REST	SETS	REPS	WEIGHT	REST	SETS	REPS	WEIGHT	REST	SETS	REPS	WEIGHT	REST

CARDIO:	TIME	DIST.	INT.	PACE	TIME	DIST.	INT.	PACE	TIME	DIST.	INT.	PACE	TIME	DIST.	INT.	PACE

WORKOUT LOG

NAME:

GOALS:

DATE:

STATS:

WEIGHT:

EXERCISE:	SETS	REPS	WEIGHT	REST	SETS	REPS	WEIGHT	REST	SETS	REPS	WEIGHT	REST	SETS	REPS	WEIGHT	REST

CARDIO:	TIME	DIST.	INT.	PACE	TIME	DIST.	INT.	PACE	TIME	DIST.	INT.	PACE	TIME	DIST.	INT.	PACE

WORKOUT LOG

NAME:

GOALS:

DATE:

STATS:

WEIGHT:

EXERCISE:	SETS	REPS	WEIGHT	REST	SETS	REPS	WEIGHT	REST	SETS	REPS	WEIGHT	REST	SETS	REPS	WEIGHT	REST

CARDIO:	TIME	DIST.	INT.	PACE	TIME	DIST.	INT.	PACE	TIME	DIST.	INT.	PACE	TIME	DIST.	INT.	PACE

WORKOUT LOG

NAME: _______________________________________

GOALS: ______________________________________

DATE: _______________________________________

STATS: ______________________________________

WEIGHT: _____________________________________

EXERCISE:	SETS	REPS	WEIGHT	REST	SETS	REPS	WEIGHT	REST	SETS	REPS	WEIGHT	REST	SETS	REPS	WEIGHT	REST

CARDIO:	TIME	DIST.	INT.	PACE	TIME	DIST.	INT.	PACE	TIME	DIST.	INT.	PACE	TIME	DIST.	INT.	PACE

WORKOUT LOG

NAME:

GOALS:

DATE:

STATS:

WEIGHT:

EXERCISE:	SETS	REPS	WEIGHT	REST	SETS	REPS	WEIGHT	REST	SETS	REPS	WEIGHT	REST	SETS	REPS	WEIGHT	REST

CARDIO:	TIME	DIST.	INT.	PACE	TIME	DIST.	INT.	PACE	TIME	DIST.	INT.	PACE	TIME	DIST.	INT.	PACE

WORKOUT LOG

NAME:
GOALS:
DATE:
STATS:
WEIGHT:

EXERCISE:	SETS	REPS	WEIGHT	REST	SETS	REPS	WEIGHT	REST	SETS	REPS	WEIGHT	REST	SETS	REPS	WEIGHT	REST

CARDIO:	TIME	DIST.	INT.	PACE	TIME	DIST.	INT.	PACE	TIME	DIST.	INT.	PACE	TIME	DIST.	INT.	PACE

WORKOUT LOG

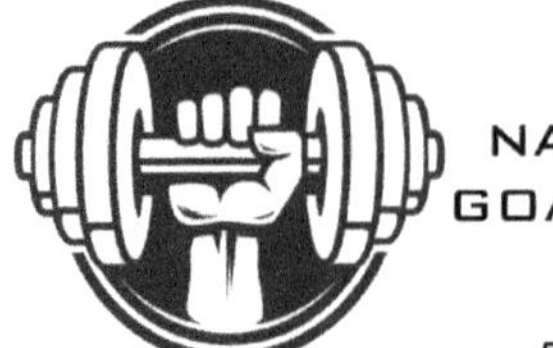

NAME:

GOALS:

DATE:

STATS:

WEIGHT:

EXERCISE:	SETS	REPS	WEIGHT	REST	SETS	REPS	WEIGHT	REST	SETS	REPS	WEIGHT	REST	SETS	REPS	WEIGHT	REST

CARDIO:	TIME	DIST.	INT.	PACE	TIME	DIST.	INT.	PACE	TIME	DIST.	INT.	PACE	TIME	DIST.	INT.	PACE

WORKOUT LOG

NAME:

GOALS:

DATE:

STATS:

WEIGHT:

EXERCISE:	SETS	REPS	WEIGHT	REST	SETS	REPS	WEIGHT	REST	SETS	REPS	WEIGHT	REST	SETS	REPS	WEIGHT	REST

CARDIO:	TIME	DIST.	INT.	PACE	TIME	DIST.	INT.	PACE	TIME	DIST.	INT.	PACE	TIME	DIST.	INT.	PACE

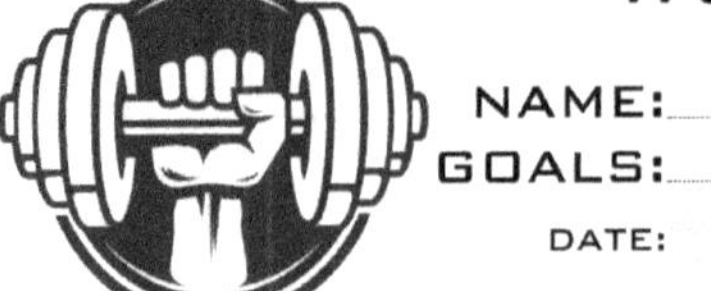

WORKOUT LOG

NAME:
GOALS:
DATE:
STATS:
WEIGHT:

EXERCISE:	SETS	REPS	WEIGHT	REST	SETS	REPS	WEIGHT	REST	SETS	REPS	WEIGHT	REST	SETS	REPS	WEIGHT	REST

CARDIO:	TIME	DIST.	INT.	PACE	TIME	DIST.	INT.	PACE	TIME	DIST.	INT.	PACE	TIME	DIST.	INT.	PACE

WORKOUT LOG

NAME:
GOALS:
DATE:
STATS:
WEIGHT:

EXERCISE:	SETS	REPS	WEIGHT	REST	SETS	REPS	WEIGHT	REST	SETS	REPS	WEIGHT	REST	SETS	REPS	WEIGHT	REST

CARDIO:	TIME	DIST.	INT.	PACE	TIME	DIST.	INT.	PACE	TIME	DIST.	INT.	PACE	TIME	DIST.	INT.	PACE

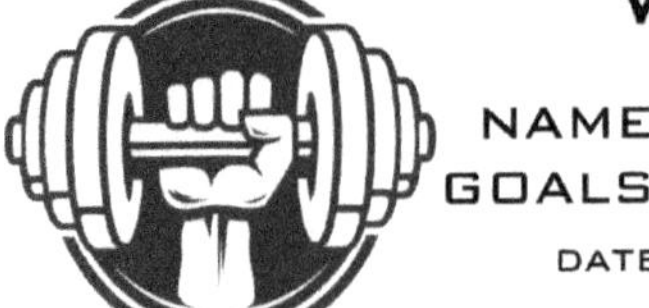

WORKOUT LOG

NAME:
GOALS:
DATE:
STATS:
WEIGHT:

EXERCISE:	SETS	REPS	WEIGHT	REST	SETS	REPS	WEIGHT	REST	SETS	REPS	WEIGHT	REST	SETS	REPS	WEIGHT	REST

CARDIO:	TIME	DIST.	INT.	PACE	TIME	DIST.	INT.	PACE	TIME	DIST.	INT.	PACE	TIME	DIST.	INT.	PACE

WORKOUT LOG

NAME:

GOALS:

DATE:

STATS:

WEIGHT:

EXERCISE:	SETS	REPS	WEIGHT	REST	SETS	REPS	WEIGHT	REST	SETS	REPS	WEIGHT	REST	SETS	REPS	WEIGHT	REST

CARDIO:	TIME	DIST.	INT.	PACE	TIME	DIST.	INT.	PACE	TIME	DIST.	INT.	PACE	TIME	DIST.	INT.	PACE

WORKOUT LOG

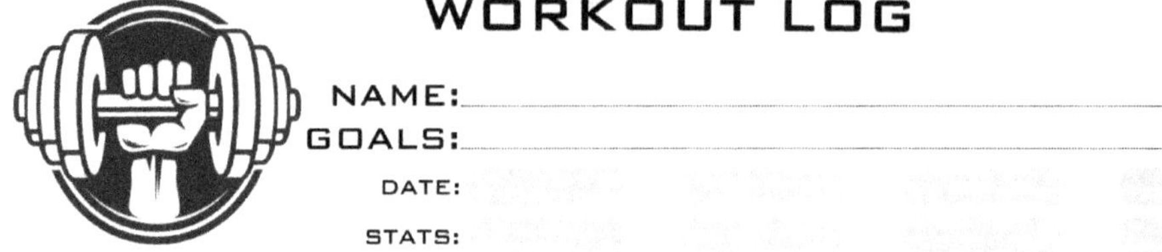

NAME:

GOALS:

DATE:

STATS:

WEIGHT:

EXERCISE:	SETS	REPS	WEIGHT	REST	SETS	REPS	WEIGHT	REST	SETS	REPS	WEIGHT	REST	SETS	REPS	WEIGHT	REST

CARDIO:	TIME	DIST.	INT.	PACE	TIME	DIST.	INT.	PACE	TIME	DIST.	INT.	PACE	TIME	DIST.	INT.	PACE

www.ingramcontent.com/pod-product-compliance
Lightning Source LLC
Chambersburg PA
CBHW070900250726
48662CB00003B/1485